GOUT CURE

No More Pain

Carl Preston

Table of Contents

Thank you!

Thank you for purchasing The Anti-Inflammatory Gout Diet! As a sign of my gratitude, I would like you to acquire my other **Anti Inflammatory Cure eBook absolutely FREE on the last page of this eBook**. No sign up for, no hassle, just plain download for you to enjoy.

Do not forget to check all the **Recipes Videos** including all the recipes of the 4-week program at the end of the Book.

Now, sit back, enjoy your read, and welcome to the path to becoming Pain Free!

Introduction

First off, we would just like to say thank you for taking the time to purchase The Anti-Inflammatory Gout Diet. This guide has been curated through personal experience and extensive additional research and planning to create the ultimate pathway to dealing with Gout once and for all. This mysterious and challenging condition can be debilitating at the best of times, and this guide will cover everything that you would possibly need to know about combatting, managing and preparing for gout in the right way.

Here is what you will get from this eBook:

- The right foods to eat.

- How to tackle the issue once and for all.

- A Detailed **4-Week meal plan** to get the reader started.

- The List of Ingredients and a How-to guide on how to Cook the **recommended meals recipes**.

- **Recipe videos** to as an extra support for you to cook the 4-Week Diet delicious recipes.

- Tips and tricks for handling gout and preserving physical condition.

- Great recipes to try out.

You might have tried medicine, you might have tried exercise – you might even have tried nothing at all. The problem with gout is that the solution to fixing it is just so simple that many people might never even consider it. What we eat directly correlates with how we feel and how we perform not just only a daily basis, but in life in general. A rather lax approach to eating properly and taking in too much of the wrong stuff can lead to a myriad range of health problems – Gout included.

Eating right, though, is a challenge many of us don't understand or know enough about to really take seriously. This makes it quite hard for people to get to grips with what they need to be doing on a daily basis, and therefore can make it very difficult for people to get the help that they need in feeling safe, feeling secure and feeling happy. We remove the significant problems that many people will suffer from with Gout and we also remove the biggest problem of the lot; the uncertainty!

With the help of this guide, you will learn everything you need to know about gout, including:

- What it is and how to beat it

- The problems it can cause

- The benefits of changing your diet and improving the way that you eat

- Changing your mindset to ensure success

- A meal plan sample

- Various recipes to put to good use when beating Gout

Everything that you could possibly need to take on Gout and do it properly is included here in this guide!

What is Gout?

To defeat any problem, you first need to know what the cause is first. Gout is something that we can suffer from without really knowing about it, and the problems that you suffer with Gout can go more or less unnoticed unless you are prepared to take the time to look around, learn about it, and take it to the next stage.

With our assistance and the information precluded in here, you will be able to take on Gout and actually deal with the problem once and for all!

So, what is Gout?

- It's a form of arthritis, whereby the crystals of sodium urate start to form both inside and around our joints.

- Gout causes a large flare-up of pain and can make the joint swell up and look extremely red.

- The symptoms can develop very quickly – within just 24 hours – and can last for up to ten day.

- Once you suffer from Gout once, you can be sure it will return in the future

What causes this to occur, then?

- Gout is caused by uric acid in the blood building up a little bit too much; it's a product we don't need yet our body makes it on a daily basis.

- The kidneys get rid of this for us, but when you produce an excess or your body gets rid (excretes) too little, you can have problems.

- This causes the build-up to start, which can occur over a period of years without your knowledge.

- The worst case scenario with gout is that the crystals in your joints start to clump and pack together, creating what is essentially a permanent level of joint damage that cannot be undone and cannot be stopped, causing immense stiffness throughout the day and making your overall day so much more challenging than it would have been previously.

What can cause Gout to start up, then?

- The older you are, the more likely it is.

- It's also four times more likely to strike in men.

- Being overweight can play a part in gout.

- Gout is a hereditary problem – it can run in the family.

- Diabetics are more likely to suffer.

- Drinking too much alcohol can also cause this to rise up.

Whilst Gout will subside in time, it will return in the future. Your best bet to stopping this process from returning is to look at how you eat; changing your diet is a proven method of prevention.

Curing Gout through Food

This book is built around the curing of Gout using food, and changing your diet to suit the needs of your body.

The problem is that eating food to manage Gout is very challenging, as you need to know exactly what you should be eating – and what you should be drinking. The good thing is that Gout-free diets are quite open and therefore you aren't subscribing to a life of bland, grey meals and boring dinners. You are subscribing to removing some dangerous and damaging foods from the menu, giving your body the right blend of things like:

- Fruits that have a darker skin like oranges, apples, cherries, peaches and blueberries can be the perfect place to get started.

- Likewise, vegetables like onion, squashes, spinach and broccoli can help you get moving alongside using things like dark, leafy greens.

- Soy products can be a good addition in small doses, too, thanks to their antioxidant qualities.

- Mushrooms like oysters are high in anti-inflammatory capabilities, which is what we need.

- Protein such as organic chicken and/or grass-fed beef products are a good way of getting inflammation.

- Raw-milk dairy products should be used if you have to.

- Try and eat as many acai berries and blueberries as you can, by the way; they are two of the most powerful anti-inflammatories on the planet, bar none!

- Go for spices like turmeric, too. Hey can be very powerful for helping you get to grips with what you need quickly and also adding extra life and flavor to meals.

- However, go for omega-3 enriched eggs if you want to have an egg.

- Red, black and kidney beans are a good addition to have in there but make sure you don't overload as you can go overboard with protein by doing this.

- Healthy fats as well as oils can be a useful source of the right ingredients to battle back against inflammation and also to provide your body with antioxidant content. Consider olive oil a bit of a staple in this thanks to it polyphenol count .

- Salmon and fatty fish are a good source of omega-3 fatty acids, too!

- If you need a bit of chocolate, make sure its dark chocolate; it's so much better for you – try and get raw cacao chocolate if you can.

When it comes to drinks, you should try and concentrate on things such as:

- Green teas if you need a drink of this caliber – the richer the better!

- Coffee is also acceptable if you want a cup, just make it black.

- Need a drink? A glass of red wine will need to be the best it gets for you, but for wine fans this can be a real punch-the-air moment!

- Pure fruit juice ideally diluted with water.

- Water, obviously!

- Semi-skimmed milk if you need to use it.

- Avoid soda and the like, however!

As you can see, this is not going to restrict you by too much. There is a fair amount on here that you might be eating anyway, but it's basically removing all the things that you eat that you don't see included within this list! The range of foods that can cause Gout and Gout attacks are quite large, so make sure that when you look at diets and foods that they fall roughly into this category.

What to Avoid

To start off with, you need to know what makes Gout so dangerous and what can make it such a serious challenge for someone who is suffering. If you aren't sure what can cause Gout, though, it can be hard to know what to take off the table so that you can eat properly and sensible. To do this, you need to look at the following foods as perfect examples of what to avoid:

- Scallops are a common source of Gout attacks, due to the fact it's loaded with purine. If you have too much purine in your diet it can cause the acid buildup to be simply too much for your body to deal with effectively.

- Herrings are another choice tory and avoid. In fact, try and avoid anchovies and tuna should be avoided as they can cause a variety of Gout symptoms to start flaring up.

- Red meats can be a bit of a problem – white meat tends to be a better choice for you. Red meat is OK if you are just dealing with something simple and you only eat it once in a blue moon.

- If you tend to eat a lot of pork or beef, you might need to cut back a little bit as they are just as bad as the above meats.

- A beer is probably not the best idea for those with Gout, sorry drinkers! This will make it hard for you to find something new to drink but, as suggested above, wine is a good leveler as it has nothing like the problems for your uric acid levels.

- Soda should always be avoided from now on – it simply does you more harm than it would ever do you good. Downing these drinks will help you gain weight really fast for a start; but they also make your body produce an excess of uric acid that causes significant problems.

- Asparagus might seem a good idea but it's not something that you would want to eat too much as they are high in purine. The odd bit is not a problem again, but if you want to eat them regularly you will be in for a bit of a shock along the way, most likely!

- Veggie-rich diets will help clear purines from the body but eating too may high-purine ones will just counteract any good work that you have done.

- Avoid eating Liver if you can; it's not very good for you in this sense as they just cause serious problems for Gout sufferers. In fact, all organ meats should be more or less avoided due to the excess strain that they can put on your system without even trying.

In short, there is plenty to try and avoid. As a rule, anything high in purine should be avoided as they tend to be the biggest inhibitors for those who are dealing with an issue lie this. Take the time that's needed to do some further research on foods that you like specifically, as it can really benefit you to know what you can and cannot take along the way.

This is just a start of the list, though, so keep on looking until you find something that you are not sure about; avoiding the bad stuff is as important as eating the right stuff when you embark on this journey.

The Benefits

There are multiple benefits to taking on this kind of lifestyle choice/diet, with the main one obviously being that you will greatly reduce the probability of a Gout attack occurring.

By sticking to what is listed above as a general rule – and you can do a bit more research yourself into individual foods you might be interested in trying, but aren't sure if they are compatible – you can start to see a whole range of benefits with your body and with your system in general. This will include things such as:

- You'll open up your palette – with the inclusion of new spices and the like (especially turmeric) you can start to really try out new meals and new combinations about way from gout-causing trash like takeout food.

- Greater flexibility – the best thing about using this solution is that the level of flexibility you will end up with is much improved over the old level that you would have had in the past. This is very important, as you will be able to be more active and more mobile without the pain and the stress of Gout holding you back.

- Give your body more nutrition – by using this diet you invariably start to make a big change to the strength of your bodies overall function. Instead of being stuck eating the same rubbish time and time again, you will now be introducing new nutrients and additional solutions into your body.

- Reduce inflammation – much like other popular diet out there that deal with inflammation, this works as an anti-inflammatory diet as you are taking in so many antioxidants and nutrients you didn't in the past. This lets your body relax and cool down a bit, and also gives you a chance to fight off inflammation that isn't caused by Gout as a nice little byproduct.

- Remove chronic pain – no longer will you need to put up with your body being in a world of pain and agony as you try and work through the day, thanks to the range of changes that are brought to the table with the help of this diet. You'll remove the struggle and the stress that so many suffer from.

The first thing that you will notice when you start eating this diet, though, is that your taste in food will change. As you start trying things that were seen as "weird" or overly nu-age in the age, you will start to appreciate the variety of food and the style of meals that you can eat as opposed to repetition in the food that you eat from time to time.

Now, let's take a look at a sample of what a week of eating a Gout-style eating plan would be made up of. You might be surprised to see that this can be quite varied and fun, as opposed to many overly restrictive diets!

FOUR-Week Meal Plan

As you obviously will know by now, your diet is going to be changing – and changing quite dramatically. We've look around online and found the best way for you to get the right kind of meals and the right kind of planning put together for your first week of eating. Since this is a long-term diet and not something you can really plan week to week in a guide, or have a specific date to follow it until, this is just an example. Every week should be different and varied, and you should now start spending time looking at new recipes and ideas that you can try.

Don't worry, we haven't let you all alone! After this page, you will find some excellent recipes that you can try out as well as great resources to go and look at if you want to really start benefiting from this kind of lifestyle change. The best thing about each meal included below is that each of them can be booked to your own style; just look up a recipe that you find online that works best for you, because these meals are always subject to your own tastes. After this you will find the cookbook with all the recipes for you to cook them easily and to enjoy them!

Just remember to avoid any recipes that use the kind of things we suggest that you avoid, for maximum results.

The Four-Week Meal Plan

Week 1

Day	Breakfast	Lunch	Dinner
Monday	Quinoa Porridge	Pumpkin Soup	Poached Egg /w veg
Tuesday	Gingerbread Oatmeal	Chicken Wraps /w your choice of smart topping	Hemp Hummus
Wednesday	Raspberry Green Tea Smoothie	Kipper Salad	Turkey Chilli
Thursday	Quinoa Granola	Sweet Potato Soup	Steamed Salmon /w Lemon Zucchini
Friday	Ginger Apple Muffins	Persimmon & Pear Salad	Pepper and Turkey Pasta
Saturday	Strawberry Crepes (avoid gluten versions!)	Lentil Soup	Quinoa /w Turkey Stuffed Peppers
Sunday	Fruit Green Tea Smoothie of your choice	Smoked Trout Tartine	Sweet Potato & Black Bean Burger

Week 2

Day	Breakfast	Lunch	Dinner
Monday	Baked oatmeal	Polenta lasagna	Jamaican Rice and Peas
Tuesday	Breakfast casserole	Vegetarian chili	Bean Burger
Wednesday	Frittata with low fat cheese	Lentil meatloaf	Lentil burger
Thursday	Roasted Garlic Cauliflower Soup	Greek white beans in tomato sauce	Felafel with tahini & tzatziki
Friday	Hummus with veggies	Spicy corn & black bean salad	Watermelon-Pineapple-Ginger Juice
Saturday	Broccoli Souffle	Gazpacho	Creamy polenta with ratatouille
Sunday	Pomegranate Smoothie	Jamaican Rice and Peas	Veggie Terrines

Week 3

Day	Breakfast	Lunch	Dinner
Monday	Cornflakes, Low-Fat Milk and berries	Vegetarian chili	Salsa chicken burritos
Tuesday	Raspberry tarts	Balsamic chicken	Rice with vermicelli
Wednesday	Warm Eggplant and Goat Cheese Sandwiches	Rosemary roasted potatoes	Lemon dill salmon
Thursday	Vanilla bean pudding	Lemon and sage roasted chicken	Orange and Duck Confit Salad
Friday	Peaches with berry sauce	Zucchini Spaghetti	Potato frittata
Saturday	Tomato crostini	Honey mustard chicken	Balsamic Chicken
Sunday	Pumpkin pancakes	Beef Stew	Vanilla Fruit Salad

Week 4

Day	Breakfast	Lunch	Dinner
Monday	Pumpkin pancakes	Gazpacho	Lemon dill salmon
Tuesday	Vanilla bean pudding	Jamaican Rice and Peas	Orange and Duck Confit Salad
Wednesday	Pumpkin pancakes	Vegetarian Chili	Lemon dill salmon
Thursday	Breakfast casserole	Lemon and sage roasted chicken	Orange and Duck Confit Salad
Friday	Frittata with low fat cheese	Zucchini Spaghetti	Lemon and sage roasted chicken
Saturday	Baked oatmeal		Zucchini Spaghetti
Sunday	Hummus with Veggies	Honey mustard chicken	Rice with Vermicelli

As you can see, this is a simple and easy menu that can be adjusted and made to suit your own tastes. We deliberately left this fairly open so that you will be anxious to go and look at new menu ideas and new solutions yourself, instead of just relying upon the same old routine week-after-week.

This is just a sample of what you can have; this diet, if you will, is all about experimentation and being willing to try out something new. Don't be afraid to let your taste buds run wild and try out something fresh and new; always try to give them something exciting and something engaging that you can experiment with and try something unique with. Got an old favorite that ticks the boxes? Then mess around and see what else you can do with an old classic!

COOKBOOK AND RECIPES

Greek white beans in tomato sauce

INGREDIENTS

- 1 lb (450 g) dried large white beans (such as gigantes, lima or cannellini)
- 1 tbsp (15 mL) + 1/4 cup (60 mL) extra-virgin olive oil
- 2 medium yellow onions, finely diced
- 4 cloves garlic, minced
- 2 large tomatoes, grated or pureed, or 2 cups (500 mL) canned crushed tomatoes
- 5.5-oz (156-mL) can tomato paste
- Kosher salt + freshly ground black pepper
- Chopped flat-leaf parsley (optional)

DIRECTIONS

1. Place beans in a large bowl. Cover with several inches water. Let stand on counter overnight. Drain; rinse.
2. Place in a large pot and fill with water. Bring to a boil over high heat. Reduce heat to medium and simmer briskly until just tender but not soft, splitting or mushy, about 30 to 60 minutes depending on the size and age of beans.
3. Drain; rinse. Transfer to ovenproof pot or casserole dish.
4. Meanwhile, heat 1 tbsp (15 mL) oil in a large skillet over medium. Add onion and garlic. Cook, stirring, 10 minutes to soften without browning. Add tomatoes and tomato paste. Season to taste with salt and pepper. Simmer over medium heat 10 minutes to thicken slightly. Stir into beans along with remaining ¼ cup (60 mL) oil.
5. Bake, uncovered, in preheated 350F (180C) oven until beans are tender and sauce has thickened, about 45 minutes. Let stand 10 minutes before serving. If desired, garnish with parsley.

Spicy corn & black bean salad

INGREDIENTS

- 4 cups corn kernels
- 1 1/2 tablespoons fajita seasoning
- 1/2 teaspoon ground black pepper
- 1 (15 ounce) can black beans, drained and rinsed
- 1 red bell pepper, chopped
- 1/2 cup chopped green onion
- 1/4 cup chopped fresh cilantro
- 1/4 cup fresh lime juice
- 2 tablespoons orange juice

DIRECTIONS

1. Heat olive oil in a large skillet over medium heat. Cook and stir corn, fajita seasoning, and black pepper in the hot oil until corn is lightly browned, 6 to 8 minutes. Remove from heat and set aside to cool.
2. Mix corn mixture, black beans, red bell pepper, green onion, jalapeno pepper, cilantro, lime juice, orange juice, and salt together in a bowl; cover and refrigerate at least 1 hour before serving.

Hummus with veggies

INGREDIENTS

- 3/4 cup mixed vegetables, such as baby carrots, cherry tomatoes and red bell pepper slices
- 3 tablespoons prepared hummus

DIRECTIONS

1. Wash vegetables and a slice them into bitable sizes
2. Arrange them on a platter
3. Dip vegetables into hummus.

Vegetarian chili

INGREDIENTS

- 2 tablespoons extra-virgin olive oil
- 1 medium yellow onion, diced medium
- 4 garlic cloves, roughly chopped
- 1 1/2 teaspoons ground cumin
- 1 teaspoon chipotle chile powder
- Coarse salt and ground pepper
- 1 medium zucchini, cut into 1/2-inch dice
- 3/4 cup (6 ounces) tomato paste
- 1 can (15.5 ounces) black beans, rinsed and drained
- 1 can (15.5 ounces) pinto beans, rinsed and drained
- 1 can (14.5 ounces) diced tomatoes with green chiles
- 1 can (14.5 ounces) diced tomatoes

DIRECTIONS

1. In a large pot, heat oil over medium-high. Add onion and garlic; cook, stirring frequently, until onion is translucent and garlic is soft, about 4 minutes.
2. Add cumin and chile powder, season with salt and pepper, and cook until spices are fragrant, 1 minute.
3. Add zucchini and tomato paste; cook, stirring frequently, until tomato paste is deep brick red, 3 minutes.
4. Stir in black beans, pinto beans, and both cans diced tomatoes.
5. Add 2 cups water and bring mixture to a boil. Reduce to a medium simmer and cook until zucchini is tender and liquid reduces slightly, 20 minutes.
6. Season with salt and pepper.

Creamy polenta with ratatouille

INGREDIENTS

- Olive Oil
- 1 medium onion, diced
- several sprigs fresh oregano or marjoram (or 1 teaspoon dried)
- 1 sprig fresh rosemary (or 1/2 teaspoon dried)
- 2-3 garlic cloves, minced
- 4 cups eggplant peeled and cubed
- 2 cups diced pepper (red, orange, yellow or green)
- 4 cups peeled and seeded tomatoes, chopped
- 1/2 teaspoon dried turmeric
- 1 bay leaf
- handful of fresh basil, chopped
- I pack instant polenta

DIRECTIONS

1. Assemble all ingredients
2. Prepare eggplant: peel and cube, place in colander
3. Sprinkle with salt and let drain for 15-20 minutes while you chop and measure the other ingredients.
4. This is not an essential step, but it releases excess water from the eggplant, making it firmer and meatier.
5. Heat a large skillet over medium high heat. When hot, add 1-2 tablespoons olive oil and sauté the onions 5-6 minutes until they start to brown on the edges.
6. Add garlic and continue to sauté for another minute.
7. Add eggplant and peppers, cook until they just begin to soften.
8. Add remaining ingredients, except the basil, stir gently, cover and reduce heat to a simmer.
9. Cook for 20-25 minutes until vegetables are tender and flavors have come together.
10. Add fresh chopped basil and combine – ready to serve
11. Cook polenta until soft
12. Add more liquid to make it creamier
13. Add grated parmesan
14. Serve ratatouille over polenta with extra basil and parmesan

Baked oatmeal

INGREDIENTS
- 2 cups/7 oz/200 g rolled oats
- 1/2 cup/2 oz/60 g walnut pieces, toasted and chopped
- 1/3 cup/2 oz/60 g natural cane sugar or maple syrup, plus more for serving
- 1 teaspoon aluminum-free baking powder
- 1 1/2 teaspoons ground cinnamon
- Scant 1/2 teaspoon fine-grain sea salt
- 2 cups/475 ml milk
- 1 large egg
- 3 tablespoons unsalted butter, melted and cooled slightly
- 2 teaspoons pure vanilla extract
- 2 ripe bananas, cut into 1/2-inch/1 cm pieces
- 1 1/2 cups/6.5 oz/185 g huckleberries, blueberries, or mixed berries

DIRECTIONS
1. Preheat the oven to 375°F/190°C with a rack in the top third of the oven. Generously butter the inside of an 8-inch/20cm square baking dish.
2. In a bowl, mix together the oats, half the walnuts, the sugar, if using, the baking powder, cinnamon, and salt.
3. In another bowl, whisk together the maple syrup, if using, the milk, egg, half of the butter, and the vanilla.
4. Arrange the bananas in a single layer in the bottom of the prepared baking dish.
5. Sprinkle two-thirds of the berries over the top.
6. Cover the fruit with the oat mixture.
7. Slowly drizzle the milk mixture over the oats. Gently give the baking dish a couple thwacks on the countertop to make sure the milk moves through the oats. Scatter the remaining berries and remaining walnuts across the top.
8. Bake for 35 to 45 minutes, until the top is nicely golden and the oat mixture has set.
9. Remove from the oven and let cool for a few minutes.
10. Drizzle the remaining melted butter on the top and serve.
11. Sprinkle with a bit more sugar or drizzle with maple syrup if you want it a bit sweeter.

Breakfast casserole

INGREDIENTS

- Nonstick cooking spray
- I pound ground maple pork sausage
- 6 slices soft hearty white bread
- One 8-ounce package shredded triple cheddar cheese
- 8 large eggs
- 2 cups whole milk
- 1 teaspoon dry mustard
- ¼ teaspoon salt
- ½ teaspoon seasoned pepper

DIRECTIONS

1. Preheat the oven to 350 degrees F. Spray a 13-by 9-inch baking sheet with nonstick cooking spray.
2. In a large skillet, cook the sausage over medium heat, stirring frequently, until brown and crumbly, about 10 minutes; drain well on paper .
3. Cut and discard the crust of the bread. Cut the slices in half, and arrange in a single layer in the prepared baking dish, cutting pieces to fit as necessary to cover the bottom of the dish.
4. Sprinkle with the sausage and cheese.
5. In a large bowl, whisk together the eggs, milk, mustard, seasoned and pepper; carefully pour the mixture over the cheese.
6. Bake casserole until set and golden, about 40 minutes.
7. Let stand for 10 minutes before serving .

Gazpacho

INGREDIENTS

- 1 hothouse cucumber. halved and seeded, but not peeled
- 2 red bell peppers, cored and seeded
- 4 plum tomatoes
- 1red onion
- 2 garlic cloves, minced
- 23 ounces tomato juice (3 cups)
- ¼ cup white wine vinegar
- ¼ cup good olive oil
- ½ tablespoon kosher salt
- 1 teaspoons freshly ground black pepper

DIRECTIONS

1. Roughly chop the cucumbers, bell peppers, tomatoes, and red onions into 1-inch cubes.
2. Put each vegetable separately into a food processor fitted with a steel blade and pulse until it is coarsely chopped. Do not overprocess!
3. After each vegetable is processed, combine them in a large bowl and add the garlic, tomato juice, vinegar, olive oil, salt, and pepper.
4. Mix well and chill before serving.
5. The longer gazpacho sits, the more the flavors develop

INGREDIENTS

For the Tzatziki
- 7 ounces Greek Yogurt
- 1/2 cup peeled and diced seedless cucumber
- 1 tablespoon lemon juice
- 1 garlic clove
- 1/2 teaspoon salt
- 1/4 teaspoon dried mint
- pinch of black pepper

For the Tahini Sauce
- 1/3 cup tahini paste
- 1/2 lemon juice
- 3 tablespoons water
- salt and pepper to taste

For the Falafel Bugers:
- 2 cans chickpeas, drained
- 1 small red onion
- 3 tablespoons flour
- 4 cloves garlic
- 1 tablespoon cumin
- 1 tablespoon chili powder
- 1 tablespoon coriander
- 1 teaspoon turmeric
- 1 teaspoon salt
- 3-4 tablespoons olive oil, divided
- 4 Rolls
- Tomatoes
- sliced cucumber
- Other toppings ideas: Lettuce, Red Onion, Feta, Kalamata Olives

DIRECTIONS

For the Tzatziki
1. Mix all ingredients together and set aside.

For the Tahini Sauce
1. Mix all ingredients together and set aside.

For the Falafel Bugers
1. Add the chickpeas, onion, garlic, flour, and spices (cumin, chili powder, coriander, tumeric, and salt) into the food processor and pulse until combined (add additional flour until it holds together).
2. Divide mixture into equal sized patties
3. Heat 1-2 tablespoons of olive oil in a large non-stick skillet over medium-high heat.
4. Add two falafel patties to the pre-heated skillet and cook for 4 minutes.
5. Gently flip patties (they are fragile!), and cook for an additional 4 minutes.
6. Remove from skillet and set aside (either keep in a warm oven or under some aluminum foil).
7. Add the remaining olive oil and repeat process with remaining 2 patties.
8. To serve: toast up buns for a few minutes under the broiler. Spread some tahini sauce on the bottom bun and top with a falafel patty. Top with desired toppings followed by a dallop of tzatziki. Serve while hot!

Roasted Garlic Cauliflower Soup

INGREDIENTS

- 1 large head cauliflower (about 2 1/2 lb.)
- 4 1/2 teaspoons olive oil
- 1 1/2 teaspoons kosher salt, divided
- 3 garlic cloves, unpeeled
- 3 cups reduced-sodium chicken broth
- 1 cup 2% reduced-fat milk
- 1/2 cup grated Manchego or Parmesan cheese
- Freshly ground black pepper
- Garnishes: olive oil, pomegranate seeds, fresh thyme leaves

DIRECTIONS

1. Preheat oven to 425°. Cut cauliflower into 2-inch florets; toss with olive oil and 1/2 tsp. salt. Arrange florets in a single layer on a jelly-roll pan. Wrap garlic cloves in aluminum foil, and place on jelly-roll pan with cauliflower.
2. Bake at 425° for 30 to 40 minutes or until cauliflower is golden brown, tossing cauliflower every 15 minutes.
3. Transfer cauliflower to a large Dutch oven. Unwrap garlic, and cool 5 minutes. Peel garlic, and add to cauliflower. Add stock, and bring to a simmer over medium heat; simmer, stirring occasionally, 5 minutes. Let mixture cool 10 minutes.
4. Process cauliflower mixture, in batches, in a blender until smooth, stopping to scrape down sides as needed.
5. Return cauliflower mixture to Dutch oven; stir in milk, cheese, and remaining 1 tsp. salt. Cook over low heat, stirring occasionally, 2 to 3 minutes or until thoroughly heated. Add pepper to taste.

Bean Burger

INGREDIENTS

- **2** cans (15.5 ounces each) black, white, or pinto beans or black-eyed peas
- **1** cup dried breadcrumbs
- **2** large eggs, lightly beaten
- **1** teaspoon coarsely ground black pepper
- **1/2** teaspoon garlic powder
- Extra Flavorings (see Burger options)
- **6** good-quality hamburger buns

DIRECTIONS

1. Drain 1 can of beans, reserving the liquid, and mash the beans in a medium bowl.
2. Drain the second can, add to the bowl with the breadcrumbs, eggs, pepper, and garlic powder.
3. Stir in Extra Flavorings if using. If necessary, add a little of the bean liquid until the mixture holds together but is not wet.
4. Divide into 6 equal portions and shape into 4-inch patties.
5. Warm the buns in a 300 degree F oven for about 5 minutes.
6. Meanwhile, heat % cup olive or canola oil in a large (12-inch) skillet over medium-high heat.
7. Add the patties and cook, turning only once, until a crisp brown crust forms on both sides, about 6 minutes total.
8. If you've chosen a burger that gets topped with cheese, add it now. Cover the skillet, turn the heat to low, and let the burgers continue to cook until the cheese melts. Top the burgers as desired

Frittata with low fat cheese

INGREDIENTS

- 8 eggs
- 2 tablespoons finely chopped fresh oregano
- 1/2 teaspoon salt
- 1/4 teaspoon freshly ground pepper
- 2 tablespoons extra-virgin olive oil
- 1 cup sliced red bell pepper
- 1 bunch scallions, trimmed and sliced
- 1/2 cup crumbled goat cheese

DIRECTIONS

1. Position rack in upper third of oven; preheat broiler.
2. Whisk eggs, oregano, salt and pepper in a medium bowl. Heat oil in a large, ovenproof, nonstick skillet over medium heat. Add bell pepper and scallions and cook, stirring constantly, until the scallions are just wilted, 30 seconds to 1 minute.
3. Pour the egg mixture over the vegetables and cook, lifting the edges of the frittata to allow the uncooked egg to flow underneath, until the bottom is light golden, 2 to 3 minutes. Dot the top of the frittata with cheese, transfer the pan to the oven and broil until puffy and lightly golden on top, 2 to 3 minutes. Let rest for about 3 minutes before serving. Serve hot or cold!

Polenta lasagna

INGREDIENTS

- 1 (26-ounce) jar marinara sauce, divided
- 1 teaspoon olive oil
- 1 cup finely chopped onion
- 1/2 cup chopped red bell pepper
- 1 cup meatless fat-free sausage, crumbled (such as Lightlife Gimme Lean)
- 1 cup chopped mushrooms
- 1/2 cup chopped zucchini
- 2 garlic cloves, minced
- 1 (16-ounce) tube of polenta, cut into 18 slices
- 1/2 cup (2 ounces) preshredded part-skim mozzarella cheese

DIRECTIONS

1. Preheat oven to 350°.
2. Spoon 1/2 cup marinara sauce into an 8-inch square baking dish to cover bottom, and set aside.
3. Heat oil in a large nonstick skillet over medium-high heat. Add onion and bell pepper; sauté 4 minutes or until tender. Stir in sausage; cook 2 minutes. Add mushrooms, zucchini, and garlic; sauté 2 minutes or until mushrooms are tender, stirring frequently. Add remaining marinara sauce; reduce heat, and simmer 10 minutes.
4. Arrange 9 polenta slices over marinara in baking dish, and top evenly with half of vegetable mixture. Sprinkle 1/4 cup of cheese over vegetable mixture; arrange remaining polenta over cheese. Top polenta with the remaining vegetable mixture, and sprinkle with remaining 1/4 cup cheese.
5. Cover and bake at 350° for 30 minutes. Uncover and bake an additional 15 minutes or until bubbly. Let stand 5 minutes before serving.

Lentil burger

INGREDIENTS

- 1 large clove garlic, peeled
- 1/4 teaspoon kosher salt
- 1/2 cup walnuts, toasted (see Tips)
- 2 slices whole-wheat sandwich bread, crusts removed, torn into pieces
- 1 tablespoon chopped fresh marjoram or 1 teaspoon dried
- 1/4 teaspoon freshly ground pepper
- 1 1/2 cups cooked or canned (rinsed) lentils (see Tips)
- 2 teaspoons Worcestershire sauce, vegetarian or regular
- 3 teaspoons canola oil, divided
- 4 whole-wheat hamburger buns, toasted
- 4 pieces leaf lettuce
- 4 slices tomato or jarred roasted red pepper
- 4 thin slices red onion

DIRECTIONS

1. Coarsely chop garlic; sprinkle with salt and mash to a paste with the side of the knife. Coarsely chop walnuts in a food processor.
2. Add bread, marjoram, pepper and the garlic paste; process until coarse crumbs form.
3. Add lentils and Worcestershire; process until the mixture just comes together in a mass. Form into four 3-inch patties (about 1/3 cup each).
4. Heat 2 teaspoons oil in a large nonstick skillet over medium heat. Cook the patties until browned on the bottom, 2 to 4 minutes.
5. Carefully turn over; reduce heat to medium-low. Drizzle the remaining 1 teaspoon oil around the burgers and cook until browned on the other side and heated through, 4 to 6 minutes more.
6. Serve on buns with lettuce, tomato (or red pepper) and onion.

Broccoli Souffle

INGREDIENTS

- 3 cups frozen chopped broccoli, thawed and drained
- 2 tablespoons butter
- 2 tablespoons all-purpose flour
- ½ teaspoon salt
- ½ cup milk
- ¼ cup grated Parmesan cheese

DIRECTIONS

1. In a saucepan over medium heat, cook and stir broccoli and butter until the butter is melted. Set 2 tablespoons broccoli aside for topping. Add flour and salt to the remaining broccoli; stir until blended. Gradually add milk. Bring to a boil; cook and stir for 2 minutes or until thickened. Remove from the heat; add cheese, stirring until cheese is melted.
2. In a large bowl, beat egg yolks until thickened and lemon-colored, about 5 minutes. Add broccoli mixture and set aside. In a small bowl, beat egg whites until stiff peaks form; fold into broccoli mixture.
3. Pour into an ungreased 1-1/2-qt. deep round baking dish. Bake, uncovered, at 350° for 20 minutes. Sprinkle with the reserved broccoli. Bake 10 minutes longer or until a knife inserted near the center comes out clean

Lentil meatloaf

INGREDIENTS

Loaf
- 1 cup dry lentils (use green/brown)
- 2 1/2 cups water or vegetable broth
- 3 tablespoons flaxseed meal (ground flaxseeds)
- 1/3 cup water (6 tablespoons)
- 2 tablespoons olive oil for sauteing **or** steam saute using 1/4 cup water
- 3 garlic cloves, minced
- 1 small onion, finely diced
- 1 small red bell pepper, finely diced
- 1 carrot, finely diced or grated
- 1 celery stalk, finely diced
- 3/4 cup oats (I used GF oats)
- 1/2 cup oat flour or finely ground oats (any flour of choice will work here too)
- 1 heaping teaspoon dried thyme
- 1/2 heaping teaspoon cumin
- 1/2 teaspoon each garlic powder & onion powder...for good measure!
- 1/4 – 1/2 teaspoon ground chipotle pepper, optional
- cracked pepper & sea salt to taste

Glaze
- 3 tablespoons organic ketchup
- 1 tablespoon balsamic vinegar
- 1 tablespoon pure maple syrup

DIRECTIONS

1. Rinse lentils. In large pot add 2 1/2 cups water with lentils. Bring to a boil, reduce heat, cover and simmer for about 40 minutes, stirring occasionally. It's ok if they get mushy, we are going to roughly puree 3/4 of the mixture when cooled. Once done, remove lid and set aside to cool (do not drain), they will thicken a bit upon standing, about 15 minutes is good.

2. Preheat oven to 350 degrees.

3. In small bowl combine flaxseed meal and 1/3 cup water, set aside for at least 10 minutes, preferably in the refrigerator. This will act as a binder and will thicken nicely upon sitting.

4. Prepare vegetables. In saute pan heat oil or water over medium heat. Saute garlic, onion, bell pepper, carrots and celery for about 5 minutes. Add spices mixing well to incorporate. Set aside to cool.

5. Using an immersion blender or food processor, blend 3/4 of the lentil mixture. For me this was an important part, I tried it other ways and this worked to help as a binder. If using an immersion blender, tilt your pot slightly to the side for easier blending. Alternately, you can mash the lentils with a potato masher or fork.

6. Combine sauteed vegetables with the lentils, oats, oat flour and flax egg, mix well. Taste, adding salt and pepper as needed, or any other herb or spice you might like. Place mixture into a loaf pan lined with parchment paper, leaving it overlapping for easy removal later. Press down firmly filling in along the edges too.

7. Prepare your glaze by combining all ingredients in a small bowl, mix until incorporated. I recommend making each tablespoon heaping so you have plenty of this great sauce on top. Spread over top of loaf and bake in oven for about 45 – 50 minutes. Let cool a bit before slicing.

Veggie Terrines

INGREDIENTS

- Kosher salt
- 8 large beet greens or ruby Swiss chard
- Butter, softened, for greasing mold
- 4 ounces/110 g cauliflower florets
- 4 ounces/110 g carrots
- 4 ounces/110 g green peas
- 1 red pepper
- 2 1/4 cups/560 ml heavy cream
- 5 eggs
- 1 1/2 ounces/40 g/1/3 cup grated Parmesan cheese
- Freshly ground black pepper

DIRECTIONS

1. Bring a large pot of water to the boil. Salt it and blanch the beet greens for 1 minute. Remove the leaves and immediately rinse under ice-cold water to set their color. Gently lay flat on tea towels, and pat dry with another tea towel. They should be completely dry.
2. Line a buttered terrine mold with a piece of parchment. Neatly lay in the beet leaves to cover the bottom and sides completely. They should dangle over the sides a bit so that they can be folded over the completed terrine later.
3. Cook the cauliflower, carrots and peas one at a time in the same pot of boiling salted water, until very tender.
4. Remove them and immediately rinse in ice-cold water to preserve their color. Drain well. Roast the pepper until very soft. Peel, seed and cut into pieces.
5. Heat the oven to 350 degrees F/180 degrees C.

Jamaican Rice and Peas

INGREDIENTS

- 1 can (19oz) Kidney beans, including liquid
- 1 can (14 oz) Coconut milk
- Water (approx 1-2/3 cups)
- 2 cloves Garlic, chopped
- 1 Small onion or 2 stalks scallion, chopped
- 1 tsp Dried thyme
- 1½ to 2 tsp Salt, to taste
- 3 tsp margarine (optional)
- 1 tsp Black Pepper
- 2 cups Long grain rice (rinsed and drained)

DIRECTIONS

1. Drain the liquid from the can of beans into a measuring cup and add the can of coconut milk and enough water to make four cups of liquid
2. Add liquid, beans, garlic, chopped onion and thyme to large pot
3. Add salt and black pepper. Bring to a boil.
4. Add rice and boil on High for 2 minutes.
5. Turn heat to Low, and cook covered until all water is absorbed (about 15 to 20 min).
6. Fluff with fork before serving.

Pomegranate Smoothie

INGREDIENTS

- 1/2 cup chilled pomegranate juice
- 1/2 cup vanilla low-fat yogurt
- 1 cup frozen mixed berries

DIRECTIONS

1. Add the juice, yogurt and berries to a blender. Cover and blend until pureed

Watermelon-Pineapple-Ginger Juice

INGREDIENTS:
- 1/3 pineapple, cored and skin removed
- 2 large watermelon slices
- 1 in (2.5 cm) piece of fresh ginger root

DIRECTIONS:
1. Cut pineapple away from core and rind.
2. Wash watermelon well and cut 2 large slices. You can juice the rind as well as the flesh of the watermelon.
3. Wash ginger root and cut a 1 in (2.5 cm) piece to juice.
4. Place all ingredients into juicer.
5. Juice.
6. Pour over ice and enjoy!

Rice with vermicelli

INGREDIENTS

- 4 Tbsp. butter
- ½ cup thin vermicelli, broken into small pieces
- 1 cup rice, rinsed
- 2¼ cups boiling water
- ¾ tsp. salt
- ¼ tsp. pepper
- ¼ tsp. cinnamon

DIRECTIONS

1. In a frying pan, melt butter then sauté vermicelli over medium/low heat, stirring often, until the pieces just begin to turn golden brown.
2. Add rice; stir-fry for further 1 minute. Stir in remaining ingredients, except cinnamon, then bring to boil.
3. Cover and cook over low heat for 12 minutes. Turn off heat; stir. Re-cover and allow to cook in own steam for 30 minutes.
4. Place on a platter, lightly sprinkle with cinnamon and serve as a side dish with vegetable stew entrees.

Warm Eggplant and Goat Cheese Sandwiches

INGREDIENTS

- 1 teaspoon olive oil
- 2 (1/4-inch) vertical slices small eggplant
- Cooking spray
- 1/4 teaspoon salt
- 1/4 teaspoon freshly ground black pepper
- 1/4 cup (2 ounces) goat cheese, softened
- 2 (1 1/2-ounce) rustic sandwich rolls
- 2 (1/4-inch) slices tomato
- 1 cup arugula

DIRECTIONS

1. Preheat oven to 275°.
2. Brush oil over eggplant.
3. Heat a large nonstick skillet coated with cooking spray over medium-high heat. Add eggplant; cook 5 minutes on each side or until lightly browned. Sprinkle with salt and pepper.
4. Spread about 1 tablespoon of goat cheese over cut side of each roll half. Place rolls on a baking sheet, cheese sides up; bake at 275° for 8 to 10 minutes or until thoroughly heated.
5. Remove from oven; top bottom half of each roll with 1 eggplant slice, 1 tomato slice, and 1/2 cup arugula. Top sandwiches with top halves of rolls.

Tomato crostini

INGREDIENTS

- 1/2 cup chopped plum tomato
- 1 tablespoon chopped fresh basil
- 1 tablespoon chopped pitted green olives
- 1 teaspoon capers
- 1/2 teaspoon balsamic vinegar
- 1/2 teaspoon olive oil
- 1/8 teaspoon sea salt
- Dash of freshly ground black pepper
- 1 garlic clove, minced
- 4 (1-inch-thick) slices French bread baguette
- Cooking spray
- 1 garlic clove, halved

DIRECTIONS

1. Preheat oven to 375º.
2. Combine first 9 ingredients.
3. Lightly coat both sides of bread slices with cooking spray; arrange bread slices in a single layer on a baking sheet. Bake at 375º for 4 minutes on each side or until lightly toasted.
4. Rub 1 side of bread slices with halved garlic; top evenly with tomato mixture.

Lemon and sage roasted chicken

INGREDIENTS

- 2 lemons, thinly sliced
- 6 fresh sage leaves
- 1 (6-pound) chicken
- 3 teaspoons olive oil, divided
- 3/4 pound parsnips, peeled and trimmed
- 3/4 pound carrots, peeled and trimmed
- 1/2 pound turnips, peeled and trimmed
- 1 pound fingerling potatoes, halved
- 2 tablespoons chopped fresh thyme

DIRECTIONS

1. Preheat oven to 425°. Place 6 lemon slices and sage leaves under skin of chicken. Put remaining lemon into cavity. Tie legs together with twine, and tuck wings under. Brush 1 teaspoon oil over chicken. Place chicken in roasting pan; roast in lower third of oven for 1 hour 15 minutes or until an instant-read thermometer registers 165°. Transfer chicken to a cutting board; let rest for 15 minutes.
2. Meanwhile, cut root vegetables into matchsticks. Toss with potatoes in a baking pan with remaining oil and thyme. Roast, stirring occasionally, for 45 minutes or until tender.
3. Remove skin from chicken. Discard lemons from cavity. Slice enough chicken to serve 4 (such as breasts), and serve with half of vegetables.

Orange and Duck Confit Salad

INGREDIENTS

- 1 tablespoon sherry vinegar
- 4 blood oranges, divided (3 sectioned, about 1 cup; 1 juiced, about 1/4 cup)
- 1 teaspoon Dijon mustard
- 1 tablespoon olive oil
- 1/4 teaspoon salt
- 1/4 teaspoon pepper
- 1 small duck confit leg (5-6 ounces), shredded, skin, fat, and bones discarded (about 3/4 cup)
- 6 cups mixed winter salad greens (such as romaine, escarole, and spinach)
- 1/4 cup skinned chopped hazelnuts, toasted

DIRECTIONS

1. In a small bowl, combine vinegar, orange juice, mustard, and oil, whisking well. Whisk in salt and pepper.
2. 2. In a large bowl, combine shredded duck, salad greens, hazelnuts, and orange sections. Drizzle with vinaigrette; serve.

Zucchini Spaghetti

INGREDIENTS

- 3 Zucchini (cut to resemble spaghetti)
- 1 1/2 cup Arugula
- 1 1/2 cups Basil Leaves
- 1/3 cup Walnuts
- 2 Garlic Cloves (smashed)
- 1/2 cup Grated Parmesan Cheese
- Olive Oil
- Salt
- Freshly Cracked Black Pepper
- Coarse Homemade Breadcrumbs (toasted, to garnish)

DIRECTIONS

1. Place the Arugula, Basil, Walnuts, Garlic and Cheese in a food processor and begin pulse. Slowly drizzle in Olive Oil and pulse until the mixture resembles a coarse paste. Season with Salt and Pepper to taste.
2. Heat a large skillet over medium-high with a few tablespoons of Olive Oil. Add the Zucchini and toss to coat in Oil.
3. Add a few tablespoons of Pesto and toss with the Zucchini. Once the Zucchini begins to take on color, transfer to a platter and top with the toasted Breadcrumbs to taste.
4. Serve warm or room temperature.
5. You may cut the Zucchini with a spiralizer, a mandolin fitted with a julienne attachment, or shaved thinly with a peeler.

Rosemary roasted potatoes

INGREDIENTS

- 1 1/2 pounds small red or white-skinned potatoes (or a mixture)
- 1/8 cup good olive oil
- 3/4 teaspoon kosher salt
- 1/2 teaspoon freshly ground black pepper
- 1 tablespoons minced garlic (3 cloves)
- 2 tablespoons minced fresh rosemary leaves

DIRECTIONS

1. Preheat the oven to 400 degrees F.
2. Cut the potatoes in half or quarters and place in a bowl with the olive oil, salt, pepper, garlic and rosemary; toss until the potatoes are well coated. Dump the potatoes on a baking sheet and spread out into 1 layer; roast in the oven for at least 1 hour, or until browned and crisp. Flip twice with a spatula during cooking to ensure even browning.
3. Remove the potatoes from the oven, season to taste, and serve.

Vanilla bean pudding

INGREDIENTS

- 2 1/2 cups 2% reduced-fat milk
- 1 vanilla bean, split lengthwise
- 3/4 cup sugar
- 3 tablespoons cornstarch
- 1/8 teaspoon salt
- 1/4 cup half-and-half
- 2 large egg yolks
- 4 teaspoons butter

DIRECTIONS

1. Place milk in a medium, heavy saucepan. Scrape seeds from vanilla bean; add seeds and bean to milk. Bring to a boil.
2. Combine sugar, cornstarch, and salt in a large bowl, stirring well. Combine half-and-half and egg yolks, stirring well. Stir egg yolk mixture into sugar mixture. Gradually add half of hot milk to sugar mixture, stirring constantly with a whisk. Return hot milk mixture to pan; bring to a boil. Cook 1 minute, stirring constantly with a whisk. Remove from heat. Add butter, stirring until melted. Remove vanilla bean; discard.
3. Spoon pudding into a bowl. Place bowl in a large ice-filled bowl for 15 minutes or until pudding cools, stirring occasionally. Cover surface of pudding with plastic wrap; chill.

Peaches with berry sauce

INGREDIENTS

- 1 cup fresh berries (blackberries, raspberries, strawberries, or a combination)
- 2 tablespoons honey
- 1 tablespoon fresh lemon juice
- 1 tablespoon Grand Marnier (optional)
- 2 peaches, pitted and sliced $
- 2 cups vanilla low-fat ice cream

DIRECTIONS

1. Combine the berries, honey, lemon juice, and Grand Marnier (if using) in a blender. Puree until smooth. Strain through a fine sieve into bowl; discard seeds and set aside.

2. Place 4 peach slices in each of 4 dessert bowls, and add 1/2 cup ice cream to each; drizzle with berry sauce.

Raspberry tarts

INGREDIENTS
- 1 cup/250 ml milk
- 1/2 vanilla bean, halved lengthwise and seeds scraped
- 3 egg yolks
- 1/4 cup/55 g sugar
- 2 tablespoons flour
- 1 tablespoon framboise (raspberry liqueur)
- 1/4 cup/60 ml heavy cream
- 1 pound/450 g fresh raspberries
- 1 (9-inch/23 cm) prepared baked cookie crust

DIRECTIONS
1. Put the milk in a saucepan. Split the vanilla bean, scraping the seeds into the milk, then drop in the pot. Heat to a simmer, remove from heat, cover, and set to infuse 10 minutes.
2. In bowl using an electric mixer, beat the yolks with the sugar until pale. Beat in the flour. Pull the vanilla bean from the milk and whisk the milk gradually into the egg mixture. Pour back into the saucepan, bring to a boil, and cook 1 minute. Remove from the heat and stir in the framboise. Strain into a bowl, cover with plastic wrap, and set aside to cool. When chilled, whip the cream and gently fold it in.
3. Spread the pastry cream evenly in the base of the prepared cookie crust. Arrange the berries neatly over top.

Pumpkin pancakes

INGREDIENTS

- 1 1⁄4 cups all-purpose flour
- 2 tablespoons sugar
- 2 teaspoons baking powder
- 1⁄2 teaspoon cinnamon
- 1⁄2 teaspoon ginger
- 1⁄2 teaspoon nutmeg
- 1⁄2 teaspoon salt
- 1 pinch clove
- 1 cup 1% low-fat milk (can be any kind)
- 6 tablespoons canned pumpkin puree
- 2 tablespoons melted butter
- 1 egg

DIRECTIONS

1. Whisk flour, sugar, baking powder, spices and salt in a bowl.
2. In a separate bowl whisk together milk, pumpkin, melted butter, and egg.
3. Fold mixture into dry ingredients.
4. Spray or grease a skillet and heat over medium heat: pour in 1/4 cup batter for each pancake.
5. Cook pancakes about 3 minutes per side. Serve with butter and syrup.
6. Makes about six 6-inch pancakes.

Cornflakes, Low-Fat Milk and berries

INGREDIENTS

- 2 cups cornflakes
- 1 cup 1% low-fat milk
- 1 cup berries, fresh or frozen, thawed

DIRECTIONS

1. Place cornflakes in a small bowl. Top with milk and berries.

Balsamic chicken

INGREDIENTS

- 4 boneless skinless chicken breast halves (see note in intro)
- 2 teaspoons lemon-pepper seasoning
- 1 1/2 teaspoons extra virgin olive oil
- 1/3 cup balsamic vinegar
- 1/4 cup chicken broth
- 2 garlic cloves, minced
- 4 teaspoons butter
- parsley sprig
- cherry tomatoes

DIRECTIONS

1. On a hard surface with meat mallet, lightly pound chicken to 1/4-inch. To minimize the mess, place the breasts/tenders in a zipper-lock bag (unsealed) before pounding (if doing so, ONLY use a flat-surface mallet -- not one with ridges).
2. Sprinkle lemon-pepper seasoning evenly on both sides of chicken. Press to adhere.
3. In a large frying pan, pour oil and heat to medium temperature.
4. Add chicken breasts and cook, turning once, about 7 minutes or until fork can be inserted in chicken with ease. If substituting tenders, cook approximately 2-3 minutes per side, or until done.
5. Remove chicken to warm serving platter (keep warm). In medium bowl, mix together vinegar, broth and garlic; add to frying pan. Cook over medium-high heat (scraping up brown meat bits) about 2-4 minutes or until mixture is reduced and syrupy.
6. Add butter; stir to melt.
7. Place chicken on serving dish and spoon sauce over chicken.
8. Garnish with parsley sprigs and cherry tomatoes.

Salsa chicken burritos

INGREDIENTS

- 2 (4 ounce) boneless skinless chicken breast halves
- 1 (4 ounce) can tomato sauce
- 1⁄4 cup salsa
- 1 (1 1/4 ounce) package taco seasoning mix
- 1 teaspoon ground cumin
- 2 garlic cloves, minced
- 1 teaspoon chili powder
- hot sauce

DIRECTIONS

1. Place chicken breasts and tomato sauce in a medium saucepan over medium high heat. Bring to a boil, then add the salsa, seasoning, cumin, garlic and chili powder. Let simmer for 15 minutes.
2. With a fork, start pulling the chicken meat apart into thin strings. Keep cooking pulled chicken meat and sauce, covered, for another 5 to 10 minutes. Add hot sauce to taste and stir together (Note: You may need to add a bit of water if the mixture is cooked too high and gets too thick.).

INGREDIENTS

- 2 tablespoons canola oil
- 1 1/2 cups chopped yellow onions
- 1 cup chopped red bell peppers
- 2 tablespoons minced garlic
- 2 to 3 serrano peppers, stemmed, seeded, and minced, depending upon taste
- 1 medium zucchini, stem ends trimmed and cut into small dice
- 2 cups fresh corn kernels (about 3 ears)
- 1 1/2 pounds portobello mushrooms (about 5 large), stemmed, wiped clean and cubed
- 2 tablespoons chili powder
- 1 tablespooon ground cumin
- 1 1/4 teaspoons salt
- 1/4 teaspoon cayenne
- 4 large tomatoes, peeled, seeded and chopped
- 3 cups cooked black beans, or canned beans, rinsed and drained
- 1 (15-ounce) can tomato sauce
- 1 cup vegetable stock, or water
- 1/4 cup chopped fresh cilantro leaves
- Cooked brown rice, accompaniment
- Sour cream or strained plain yogurt, garnish
- Diced avocado, garnish
- Essence, recipe follows, garnish
- Chopped green onions, garnish Emeril's ESSENCE Creole Seasoning (also referred to as Bayou Blast):
- 2 1/2 tablespoons paprika
- 2 tablespoons salt
- 2 tablespoons garlic powder
- 1 tablespoon black pepper
- 1 tablespoon onion powder
- 1 tablespoon cayenne pepper
- 1 tablespoon dried oregano
- 1 tablespoon dried thyme

DIRECTIONS

1. In a large, heavy pot, heat the oil over medium-high heat. Add the onions, bell peppers, garlic, and serrano peppers, and cook, stirring, until soft, about 3 minutes. Add the zucchini, corn, and mushrooms, and cook, stirring, until soft and the vegetables give off their liquid and start to brown around the edges, about 6 minutes. Add the chili powder, cumin, salt and cayenne, and cook, stirring, until fragrant, about 30 seconds. Add the tomatoes and stir well. Add the beans, tomato sauce, and vegetable stock, stir well, and bring to a boil. Reduce the heat to medium-low and simmer, stirring occasionally, for about 20 minutes.
2. Remove from the heat and stir in the cilantro. Adjust the seasoning, to taste.
3. To serve, place 1/4 cup of brown rice in the bottom of each bowl. Ladle the chili into the bowls over the rice. Top each serving with a dollop of sour cream and spoonful of avocado. Sprinkle with Essence and green onions and serve.

Lemon dill salmon

INGREDIENTS

- 4 (6-oz.) salmon fillets
- 1/2 teaspoon salt
- 1/4 teaspoon freshly ground pepper
- 8 fresh dill sprigs
- 4 lemon slices, halved

DIRECTIONS

1. Preheat oven to 425º. Place salmon fillets on a lightly greased rack on an aluminum foil-lined jelly-roll pan; sprinkle with salt and pepper. Place 2 dill sprigs and 2 lemon halves on each fillet.
2. Bake at 425° for 15 to 20 minutes or just until fish flakes with a fork.

Potato frittata

INGREDIENTS

- 3 large red potatoes, peeled and cut into 1/2-inch cubes
- 1 cup diced onion
- Salt and freshly ground black pepper
- 4 to 5 tablespoons olive oil, or to taste
- 6 large eggs
- 2 to 3 tablespoons freshly grated Locatelli-Romano
- Minced fresh parsley leaves

DIRECTIONS

1. Pat dry the potatoes and onions.
2. In a large, nonstick skillet set over moderate heat, heat 2 tablespoons of the oil until hot. Add the potatoes and salt and pepper and cook, stirring, for 1 minute. Add the onion and cook, stirring occasionally, until golden brown and just tender. Transfer to a plate.
3. In a bowl, combine the eggs, Locatelli-Romano, and salt and pepper. Add the vegetable mixture and gently stir to combine.
4. Add 1 to 2 tablespoons of oil to the skillet and heat it over moderate heat until hot. Add the vegetable and egg mixture and cook it over moderately low heat until golden brown and set on the underside. Invert a plate over the skillet and flip the frittata onto the plate.
5. Add another tablespoon of oil to the skillet and slide the frittata back in, uncooked side down. Cook until completely set.
6. Transfer to a plate and cut into wedges. Sprinkle with parsley.

Honey mustard chicken

INGREDIENTS
- 1/4 to 1/3 cup smooth Dijon mustard
- 1/4 to 1/3 cup honey
- 1 Tbsp olive oil
- 2-3 pounds chicken thighs (or legs)
- Salt
- 2 sprigs rosemary (or a generous sprinkling of dried rosemary)
- Freshly ground black pepper

DIRECTIONS
1. Preheat the oven to 350°F. In a medium bowl, whisk together the mustard, honey, and olive oil. Add a pinch of salt and taste. Add more salt and mustard until you get the flavor where you want it.
2. Salt the chicken lightly and lay the pieces skin-side up in a shallow casserole dish. Spoon the honey mustard sauce over the chicken. Place the rosemary sprigs in between the pieces of chicken.
3. Bake for 45 minutes, or until the thighs read 175° on a meat thermometer, or the juices run clear when the meat is pierced with a knife. Remove the casserole pan from the oven, use a spoon to spoon off any excess chicken fat that has rendered during the cooking.
4. Sprinkle some freshly ground black pepper over the chicken before you serve.

Vanilla fruit salad

INGREDIENTS

- 5 cans (20 ounces each) plus 1 can (8 ounces) pineapple chunks
- 4 packages (5.1 ounces each) instant vanilla pudding mix
- 8 cans (15 ounces each) mandarin oranges, drained
- 10 medium red apples, chopped

DIRECTIONS

1. Drain pineapple, reserving juice; set pineapple aside. Add enough cold water to juice to make 6 cups.
2. In a very large bowl, whisk juice mixture and pudding mix for 2 minutes. Let stand for 2 minutes or until soft-set. Stir in the oranges, apples and reserved pineapple. Refrigerate until chilled.

Beef stew

INGREDIENTS

- 1/4 cup plus 1 tablespoon all-purpose flour
- 2 teaspoons kosher salt, plus more for seasoning
- 1 teaspoon freshly ground black pepper, plus more for seasoning
- 1 (3-pound) boneless chuck roast
- 3 tablespoons vegetable oil
- 1 medium yellow onion, large dice
- 2 tablespoons tomato paste
- 1 cup dry red wine
- 4 cups (1 quart) low-sodium beef broth
- 2 bay leaves
- 4 fresh thyme sprigs
- 3 medium carrots
- 3 medium celery stalks
- 4 medium Yukon Gold potatoes (about 1 1/2 pounds)
- 1 cup frozen peas

DIRECTIONS

1. Place 1/4 cup of the flour and the measured salt and pepper in a large bowl and whisk to combine; set aside. Trim the roast of excess fat and sinew and cut it into 1- to 1-1/2-inch cubes. Place the meat in the flour mixture and toss to coat; set aside.

2. Heat the oil in a large, heavy-bottomed pot or Dutch oven over medium heat until shimmering. Shake off the excess flour from about one-third of the meat and add it to the pot. Cook, stirring rarely, until browned all over, about 4 to 5 minutes. Remove to a large bowl. Repeat with the remaining meat in 2 more batches; set aside.

3. Add the onion to the pot and season with salt and pepper. Cook, stirring occasionally, until softened and just starting to brown, about 5 minutes. Add the tomato paste, stir to coat the onion, and cook until the raw flavor has cooked off, about 1 to 2 minutes.

4. Sprinkle in the remaining tablespoon of flour and cook, stirring occasionally, until the raw flavor has cooked off, about 1 minute. Pour in the wine, scrape up any browned bits from the bottom of the pot, and cook until the mixture has thickened, about 3 minutes.

5. Return the meat and any accumulated juices in the bowl to the pot. Add the broth, bay leaves, and thyme and stir to combine. Increase the heat to high and bring to a boil. Immediately reduce the heat to low and simmer uncovered for 1 hour.

6. Cut the carrots, celery, and potatoes into large dice and add them to the pot (peel the carrots and potatoes first, if desired). Stir to combine, cover with a tightfitting lid, and simmer, stirring occasionally, until the vegetables and meat are knife tender, about 1 hour more.

7. Remove and discard the bay leaves and thyme stems. Stir in the peas and simmer uncovered until warmed through, about 5 minutes. Taste and season with salt and pepper as needed.

Useful Sources for Recipes

Having looked around online when we found ourselves trying to get into the anti-inflammatory haven that is Gout, we found that the best way to go about this was to look around online.

We've scoured the web and checked out key websites such as Health, The Gout Killer, and social media superstore Pinterest to find your some brilliant recipes that you can check out. Now, you can start looking around and finding other recipes to go on top of these brilliant solutions, helping you get yourself in the right mood for changing your diet and getting rid of Gout;

The Anti-Inflammatory Shake

This simple little guide will give you a great idea for making an awesome anti-inflammatory shake. It's a cracking snack or a great breakfast to give your body the help it needs in getting started for the day. The ingredients are incredibly simple to find, as well!

Find it here: https://uk.pinterest.com/pin/469852173603352206/

Uric Acid Remover

This simple shale from The Homestead Survival is well worth checking out, purely for the content and what it will feed your body with if you take it. It's loaded with the goodies that we need, and this ensures that you can get the help that you need in feeling spectacular permanently!

Find it here: https://uk.pinterest.com/pin/469852173603352206/

Cherry Smoothie

Another simple choice, this great little cherry smoothie will give your body a sweet overload of all the stuff that we really do need to stay at the top of our game. This is well worth looking into if you need an easy snack.

Find it here: http://thegoutkiller.com

Chicken & Veg

A real staple, this should be something that you look into as soon as possible as a solid one to have when you just want to eat and don't need anything too fancy or too engaging. It's an easy going and simple to enjoy, giving you nutritional balance.

Find it here: http://thegoutkiller.com/

Eggplant & Goat Cheese Toastie

Another one you probably would never go near normally, but this will give you plenty of extras that you will simply loving taking in. a brilliant option to get started with if you need something that's easy to get started with and simply digested.

Find it here: http://thegoutkiller.com/

Carrot, Potato & Ginger Soup

This one from Health is worth checking out for the taste alone; it's a great meal to have in that it gives you plenty of nutrition with minimal levels of purine. Not sure where to start with soup? Then you should definitely get on this.

Find it here:
http://www.health.com/health/gallery/0,,20448271_2,00.html

Finding Inspiration

One thing that you do need to look out for when you start this diet, though, is a lack of inspiration. With so much to choose from but so much to change from your old diet, getting to where you need to be in terms of understanding and appreciating food can be a long path you aren't really prepared for. To aoid this from occurring and making sure you have the best chance possible of finding the inspiration that you need, we recommend you check out the following resources for even more help in getting to grips with Gout dieting;

MyFoodHealth

This is a fantastic meal planner and diet assistant that can keep you on the right track and save you from making any silly mistakes along the way. This will detail all the things that you need to know and all of the most important aspects of looking after your health in general.

If you need help in getting prepared for this kind of thing, then you should really use a food planner; they work to specific diets and to typical forms of lifestyle and medical conditions so that you can get the tailored assistance that you need here.

Find it here: http://www.myfoodheth.com

The Perfect Combination

Not sure where to start? Then the brilliant Death to Diabetes is just what you need! It's a brilliant website loaded with all the information that you could possibly need about finding the best anti-inflammatory foods for you personally. It takes a bit of time and learning to get used to it, sure, but if you do it you will really benefit for quite some time thanks to the intricate and comfortable nature of the options provided.

Find it here: http://www.deathtodeiabetes.com

Natural Changes

Changing your diet to fight back against this kind of problem is something that you need to really work at and look out for, a falling into old habits can be an easily managed problem. However, not everyone is going to want to stop just at this for lifestyle changes and additions. Natural changes that you can make to your life to start combatting Gout normally are delivered in this video in an easy to understand format that ensures you get easy and simple knowledge of what you need to do, as well as making it easy to manage these changes later on down the line.

This brilliant list of tips from Mercola can help you see other ways to start changing your health and giving yourself a route forward in life that will maintain your health and your overall level of dependency on yourself as much as anyone else.

Find it here: http://www. http://articles.mercola.com/sites/articles/archive/2010/01/19/five-steps-to-overcoming-gout-naturally.aspx

Planning Chart

It always helps to have more information and even more advice to follow, and if you go to the guide above you will find it easy to get inspired. Mayoclinic have broken down the obvious things to think about here, and also provide yet more ideas for a menu that you could have in the morning. Follow what is provided in there and you should really start to benefit from the information that is provided to you on the chart.

If you don't know where to start with this kind of thing, we recommend checking out the above. It will make understanding the diet from a medical perspective a little easier and also give you another quick reference tool alongside this e-book to look at when you need some additional hints and tips.

Find it here: http://www. http://www.mayoclinic.org/healthy-lifestyle/nutrition-and-healthy-eating/in-depth/gout-diet/art-20048524

VIDEO RECIPES

Enjoy here the how-to make videos of all recipes needed to follow our detailed 4-week anti-Inflammatory diet plan, Enjoy them!

Quinoa Porridge: https://www.youtube.com/watch?v=fJRaNelgVGw

Pumpkin Soup: https://www.youtube.com/watch?v=cJ45xMhuhQc

Poached egg with Veg:
https://www.youtube.com/watch?v=nNbB5NHphxc

Gingerbread Oatmeal:
https://www.youtube.com/watch?v=cUUTBOpIC18

Chicken Wraps: https://www.youtube.com/watch?v=n7SPtr8LlGg

Hemp Hummus: https://www.youtube.com/watch?v=Hv_VWoim4XY

Raspberry Green Tea Smoothie:
https://www.youtube.com/watch?v=YquhDpvVUIc

Kipper Salad: https://www.youtube.com/watch?v=uEbZPzAu_yw

Turkey Chili: https://www.youtube.com/watch?v=UImk6hWP31w

Quinoa Granola: https://www.youtube.com/watch?v=UImk6hWP31w

Sweet Potato Soup:
https://www.youtube.com/watch?v=ZCwHxwRm0Cc

Steamed Salmon with Lemon Zucchini:
https://www.youtube.com/watch?v=lid2aZVgBmQ

Apple Muffins: https://www.youtube.com/watch?v=5WI4uQyChYQ

Persimmon Salad: https://www.youtube.com/watch?v=4anrQoKFD4w

Sausage and Pepper Pasta:
https://www.youtube.com/watch?v=y4JOqnNHEJ8

Strawberry Crepes: https://www.youtube.com/watch?v=m7s7rpvBthA

Lentil Soup: https://www.youtube.com/watch?v=fhFZVZU6DGg

Quinoa Stuffed Peppers:
https://www.youtube.com/watch?v=LIySHzemFo8

Fruit Green Tea Smoothie:
https://www.youtube.com/watch?v=X06mAd3ixcA

Smoked Trout: https://www.youtube.com/watch?v=zVu0uajsIuM

Sweet Potato and Black Bean Burger:
https://www.youtube.com/watch?v=sslMRNxiOn4

Baked Oatmeal: https://www.youtube.com/watch?v=VkaVTQXLA90

Polenta Lasagna: https://www.youtube.com/watch?v=q3Ulv0yZm48

Breakfast Casserole: https://www.youtube.com/watch?v=F3bztDC-pw4

Vegetarian Chili: https://www.youtube.com/watch?v=bkRNeN_Pmc4

Jamaican Rice and Peas:
https://www.youtube.com/watch?v=50lL7D2Dec8

Bean Burger: https://www.youtube.com/watch?v=OHJ5h9noNDU

Lentil Meatloaf: https://www.youtube.com/watch?v=yvKlmrAEuRw

Lentil Burger: https://www.youtube.com/watch?v=x3jKrq8xXw8

Roasted Garlic Cauliflower Soup:
https://www.youtube.com/watch?v=hRBVpWhTu5k

beans in tomato sauce:
https://www.youtube.com/watch?v=xRRQ5tvyoMo

Falafel with tahini & tzatziki:
https://www.youtube.com/watch?v=G_RFfoQ66W0

Hummus with veggies: https://www.youtube.com/watch?v=zS4OFgihG-4

spicy corn & black bean salad:
https://www.youtube.com/watch?v=YMEA3SI2IuU

Watermelon-Pineapple-Ginger Juice:
https://www.youtube.com/watch?v=5tT7CBLCVJk

Broccoli Souffle: https://www.youtube.com/watch?v=mZiYX1sczYY

Gazpacho: https://www.youtube.com/watch?v=vO_0joLyBOY

Creamy polenta with ratatouille:
https://www.youtube.com/watch?v=qwsffknoLSE

Pomegranate Smoothie:
https://www.youtube.com/watch?v=h_bzgxC31sY

Jamaican Rice and Peas: https://www.youtube.com/watch?v=-
kz0MtDMP5I

Cornflakes, Low-Fat Milk and berries:
https://www.youtube.com/watch?v=TomFarT5D2g

Salsa chicken burritos:
https://www.youtube.com/watch?v=hF_83UGyx_g

Raspberry tarts: https://www.youtube.com/watch?v=3bE2zS0qWPY

Balsamic chicken: https://www.youtube.com/watch?v=fJosb0RwLlc

Rice with vermicelli: https://www.youtube.com/watch?v=Cd3GwX9jB9g

Warm Eggplant and Goat Cheese Sandwiches:
https://www.youtube.com/watch?v=30cVVXO6PuU

Rosemary roasted potatoes:
https://www.youtube.com/watch?v=eM2qDPUE9wI

Vanilla bean pudding:
https://www.youtube.com/watch?v=01XCeOQHQGg

Lemon and sage roasted chicken:
https://www.youtube.com/watch?v=zUUnyYcWzjo

Orange and Duck Confit Salad:
https://www.youtube.com/watch?v=4vElRu-nqNo

Peaches with berry sauce:
https://www.youtube.com/watch?v=VGnUUlrhSkk

Zucchini Spaghetti: https://www.youtube.com/watch?v=xm6FJ9huK_4

Potato frittata: https://www.youtube.com/watch?v=ic70lzv6y3c

Tomato crostini: https://www.youtube.com/watch?v=U3aEulHVElA

Honey mustard chicken:
https://www.youtube.com/watch?v=r4QUHxKrsf4

Beef Stew: https://www.youtube.com/watch?v=nIK-GQ2uplg

Vanilla Fruit Salad: https://www.youtube.com/watch?v=fD5mpcDx4Rl

Conclusion

Thanks for reading **The Gout Free Diet**, we hope that you enjoyed reading it and that you were able to find some inspiration. Now you know how to combat Gout and remove the problems it brings to the table, you can start to transform your life and give yourself something a little bit different to follow later on down the line, for the rest of your life in fact!

This will help you totally alter the way that you feel about food and how you start to feel in general. New changes in this diet that are freshly introduced make a massive change to the overall psyche that you will approach wellness and health with, and you should also notice a significant drop-off in Gout problems.

By removing the inflammation and giving your body the aid that it needs, feeling better has never been easier. Use the recipes and the resources above to guide you and give yourself the help that you need in feeling the best that you can.

Follow this correctly, and you can finally say goodbye to those irritating Gout problems one and for all! Best of luck!

Thanks again!

Manufactured by Amazon.ca
Acheson, AB

13153312R00042